Mothers' Guide to Returning to Work

What to Expect Upon Returning to Work

Mothers' Guide to Returning to Work

What to Expect Upon Returning to Work

by

Evren Suri Westhead

Mothers' Guide to Returning to Work
What to Expect Upon Returning to Work
Copyright © 2016 Evren Suri Westhead

ISBN-13: 978-1523869459
ISBN-10: 1523869453

Dedication

This book is dedicated to my parents, Leyla and Mehmet. May all kids be so lucky to be surrounded by such tender hearts as yours.

Contents

Acknowledgments

I extend my sincerest thanks to Dr. Samantha Saffy who gave me the opportunity and space to work with mothers during their perinatal period. Also, to Marion Falling RCC for lending me her critical ear while encouraging me to stand my ground.

Also, as ever, my sincere love and affection goes out to my parents, who have been my number one support in life, as well as my husband, for his unwavering support in all my endeavors.

Foreword

This book has been written as a guide to help mothers plan out their return-to-work process before they go on their maternity leaves. It highlights what one can expect and prepare for before, during, and after maternity leave. Above all else, this guide should serve as a reminder that you are not alone in your experience as a mother during this time of transition. It is my deep hope that this book will provide you with some meaningful pointers to organize your life during this process.

This book is a necessity.

I have written it for all the mothers out there who believe they do not measure up. To those who believe there must be something wrong with them, that they are failing their baby as a mother, that they are not living up to their family's and friends' expectations – this book belongs to you. In the meantime, care providers will find value here, as well.

First and foremost, I intend to even out our expectations in terms of the initial months of motherhood. This period of time exists in stark contrast to the images of blissful-looking mothers we see in mother-and-baby portraits. It's rarer to encounter commentary on the real day-to-day work of motherhood, complete with how challenging it is, much less everything that one goes through to stay afloat (unless of course we are discussing postpartum depression). The accepted tones of pregnancy and motherhood tip too far toward the angelic and the peaceful. In reality, however, the initial months are *work*, and most mothers are hard-pressed to admit that they feel that motherhood is more like a chore than like bliss. So if you do not mesh with the mainstream image of a new mom, don't fret. It is time to declare that this is the norm, rather than the exception. Rather than wondering what is wrong with themselves, mothers should expect a high level of hard work, mixed with shock. This will help them to extend kindness toward themselves in their hour of confusion and hardship.

1. What Change Triggers and How You Cope

Before we talk about leaving or returning to work to take care of your new baby, it is important that we discuss some basic concepts that will be of use when you find yourself facing the challenges of those initial months of motherhood.

The mood cycles

Every big change in our lives involves a process that is very similar to grief. We leave one way of being behind, which requires us to change a great deal, only to start a whole new one, which requires us to change just as much. Having a baby is one such pivotal change in a woman's (and her whole family's) life. If you have not yet taken an inventory of your life, then spend some time considering your day-to-day reality, and how it stands to be both enriched and limited in many ways, at least in the first two years of raising a child.

Knowing the cycle of grief can be useful when it comes to recognizing the emotions and shifts that characterize all new mothers, yourself included. Note that I am calling it a "cycle" rather than a "stage" because it does not necessarily pass with stark efficiency. Rather, new moms mostly find ourselves in the eye of a storm. Some days (or moments), we feel that we have a better hang of it, are better able to cope with it, but shortly thereafter we may get discouraged, feeling like we're back where we were two weeks ago. If you find yourself in this cycle, I have three words for you: Hang in there. While you may not be able to see the end of it from where you're standing, I assure you that things do change – that is one thing we can all be certain of. You may not see quite how at first, but you will start feeling differently as time goes on.

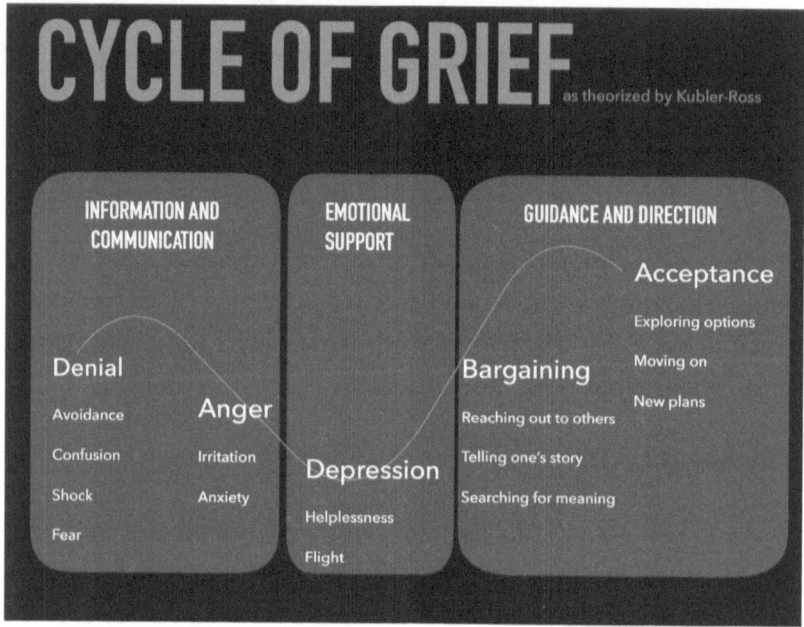

How you may face these cycles

While we are on the topic of coping, let's talk about coping strategies. Coping strategies are the behaviors, thoughts, and emotions that you use to adjust to the changes that occur in your life.

We encounter two major coping styles in the literature: problem-solving coping, which focuses on ways to tackle a given issue and/or situation in order to reduce stress, and emotion-focused coping, which consists of nurturing one's emotional health during a stressful period. In the coming chapters, I ask you to search yourself to find your dominant coping style. You will find that, consistent with the literature, your coping strategies are either active or avoidant. Active coping strategies involve an awareness of the stressor, followed by attempts to reduce the negative outcome. By contrast, avoidant coping is characterized by ignoring the issue, often resulting in activities that serve to aid in the denial of the problem (e.g., drinking, sleeping, isolating).

2. Before Going Away for Maternity Leave

Prior to initiating your maternity leave, your first step, without committing yourself one way or the other, is to learn about the various Return To Work options from your employer. If you are worried that this action might trigger some suspicion on your employer's part about your intentions after RTW, then be up front and clear about it. If you neglect to discuss the issue in advance, you will find it even harder to open the discussion later on, when you might need to most.

The truth is, you will not know for certain whether you want to go back to work or stay at home before you become a mother. Although you may have a good guess, it's wise to remain open to being surprised. The main factors that will affect your RTW decision are...

- Availability and quality of external support
- Financial ability to stay at home or hire help
- Emotional readiness to part with your baby in the daytime
- Emotional readiness to stay away from outside work

In some instances, mothers will decide to create their own schedule at work, start working from home, or start their own businesses. All these options bring with them positives and negatives to consider, chief among them their demands on your time and your resulting income security.

Above all else, the basic question that all mothers struggle with is "Am I being a good mother?" This question applies whether you are thinking, "I cannot stay at home; it will make me unhappy. Am I being a bad mother by ignoring my kids?" or "I cannot go back to work; I am unhappy there. Am I setting a bad example for my kids?"

Whatever your decision ends up being, it will consist of a balancing act.

Meanwhile, do not take the comments that get thrown back and forth in the so called "Mommy Wars" personally. It bears remembering that people lash out the most when they are conflicted within themselves, and thus trying to resolve a personal conflict.

If and when you decide to RTW, then make a strong decision to keep yourself engaged in the world of work, especially if you decide to stay away from work for more than a year. While away, you can keep up to date about changes in your industry, and even upgrade your skills through various courses. This way, you will be more comfortable accepting and talking about your off time, especially in one-year-plus situations.

Back at the workplace, make sure to maintain contact with an assigned contact person with whom you can discuss your RTW process. Ideally, this person will be directly affected by your return, as that will ensure strong/committed communication from both sides.

3. Before Returning to Work

This is the time for you and your partner to communicate your expectations to one another. What kind of free time can you give each other? Who is going to take care of which part of the daily routine, from getting the kids dressed to having breakfast in the morning to drop-offs and pickups surrounding dinners and sick days. A lot of details will need to be harmonized, and you will discover more of them over time as you go through the motions of parenthood. In order to avoid any confusion, it is advisable to start practicing your RTW routine at least two weeks before the actual return date, the better to discover and resolve any expectation issues ahead of time.

Returning to work calls for a family plan:

Becoming a mother changes a woman physically, socially, and psychologically, whether one gives birth to or adopts a child. Meanwhile, the arrival of a new baby also triggers changes, transformations, and possibly crises in the family unit. You may experience a shift in the roles or the amount of responsibility on one or both partners, and in some cases the resulting tension may reach a breaking point. More often than not, the previous approach to doing things does not meet the demands of life after the child; habits, routines, and even partners often have to transform. Likewise, issues that the family was able to manage or ignore before may become hard to overlook in these months, leading many couples to reevaluate their relationships, either openly or covertly. The good news is, these reevaluations can lead to improved circumstances.

Success is directly related to the partners' work culture:

Returning to work (RTW) is one of numerous transitions to be navigated after the arrival of a child. Many women and families, whether the mother is looking forward to returning to work or would rather stay at home yet just has to return, face the challenge of managing yet another change in routine. RTW both significantly affects and is significantly affected by the partners, along with their attitudes, to say nothing of the mother-and-baby duo. The whole family unit needs to adjust to mother's new schedule, as well as the mental strain that she will experience due to having added responsibilities. Accordingly, the success of the mother's RTW is significantly related to the positive attitude and availability of the partner. In addition, the partner's availability and involvement are directly connected to how the employer and work culture pertaining to that partner perceive his/her role. Said employers' attitude (corporate atmosphere) toward child-rearing stand to determine fathers' own length of leave and level of marital support.

After having a child, the mother's partner will often experience an increased motivation to support the family, leading to an increased engagement in work. Therefore, the workplace culture of both partners should be a key discussion point.

In the case of single mothers, they are assuming the dual role of parent and provider, and thus *require* a work culture that supports her being both a nurturing and providing role in her family unit.

Confusion about needs leads to increased emotional and strategic hardship:

The mother may indeed have conflicting ideas about whether she should return to work or stay with her baby. The confused mother (whether she stays at home or returns to work) perceives more infant distress, has a stronger tendency to take infant discontent as a personal affront, and experiences more separation anxiety than mothers who were not conflicted and planned out their return-to-work process. Therefore, it is critical that we clarify where we stand, what we want, and what we can do with the resources available to us during this transitional time. Clearing our heads about our needs and options helps us to plan and manage this process more fluently, both personally and as a family.

As a result, RTW planning *requires* the participation of both partners.

In the remainder of this chapter, we will explore some topics that may help with your exploration of and articulation on where you and your partner stand at this time. As you read on and think about how some of these issues may be pertinent to you, it is also advisable to talk them over with someone who is a friendly ear and a good listener. Most of the time, hearing ourselves articulate our ideas can provide us with clues as to our next step.

It's important to note that I'm not suggesting that mothers should think a certain way or take a certain course, but I am suggesting that you recognize whether these issues are of relevance to you. It is most favorable to take all the issues into consideration before arriving at a conclusion as to the best course.

Mothers who've interrupted their careers have several issues to consider when taking inventory of themselves. At the top of the list is the inevitable physiological and hormonal changes that continue for up to 8 months post-partum. So if you are planning to RTW earlier than 8 months, you can expect to feel as though you're not yet your usual self. Your body will still be adjusting at that time. In fact, you will not be your "usual self" even after these 8 months, because mothers' brains physically shrink during pregnancy, then regrow to help them become more apt in their new role. So that "usual self", even once reclaimed, will not entirely look the same, nor feel or think the same way about work, either, after the physical recovery is over.

Mothers very commonly worry about a diminishing mother-child relationship if and when they RTW. This concern can take the shape of not trusting the other care takers, perhaps fearing that

17

the child will bond more with them. In most cases, however, this is an unjustified fear, since kids, while they may enjoy and reciprocate others' love and attention, do not confuse the place of or place a higher value upon these relationships. Just the same, the mother's belief system and basic perception may suggest to her otherwise, which can add significant distress to the RTW process.

Meanwhile, society issues ambivalent expectations wherein one should be both a devoted and selfless care giver to her kids and also be successful in her career. Many women internalize this message and work tirelessly to accomplish such a balance, not even recognizing that this is an expectation that has been placed on them from outside. It may lead one to be proud that she can "be everywhere at once" and "do it all", but the truth is, without adequate logistical support systems to help the mother handle the high demands of both occupation and motherhood, the balance will come at a high cost. Imagine the amount of training and support medical doctors have before being handed the responsibility of caring or making decisions for human beings' lives. Well, although mothers are given the message that what they are doing is extremely delicate and important, they are also given little to no training or support, based on the assumption that they should just know how to care for this helpless little human being "naturally." To be sure, a very steep learning curve applies, making parenthood about far more than just going through the tasks.

Very frequently, mothers say how self-care or "me time" is not possible for her. Ironically, though, a mother cannot afford to *not* take care of herself, because nobody can take her place when she is not at the top of her game. More on this later.

a. Conflicting Goals

Identifying your motivations in going back to work can be very helpful when you are struggling with questions as to why you are at work or at home. Financial motives may seem the most obvious. Most everybody has some debt to pay off or some reason to save money, but when we look deeper, mothers seem to have other motivators besides money. Here is a compiled list:

- Help out with the bills
- Keep skills up to date
- Adult interaction
- Need a break from being full-time mother
- Mental health, use brain again, have fun being back
- Fulfilling workplace, employer, colleague, or client needs
- Perceived threat of losing a job
- Exploring new opportunities

Each of these points warrant at least some discussion, since they stand to illuminate your priorities and needs.

After exploring your priorities and needs, one more thing to consider is what resources are available for help. One such resource is the support of family and friends. Yet, for working couples, it's not always so simple, for reasons such as the following:

- Parents / In-laws may be far away or deceased
- Parent / In-laws may not be helpful

- Peers are usually absent/working, cannot dispel child-rearing worries
- Peers may be overly busy or at a different life stage
- Others may be judgmental about your choice to work, including fellow professionals
- Employers may doubt commitment to work (jeopardizing both childcare and room for advancement)

After one has children, life takes on a very different quality. The change is hard to understand cognitively before you have kids. You do not even quite understand it when you are pregnant. All the factors listed above, when not examined, stand a chance to catch mothers and family units off guard.

b. Exercise Your Return to Work Options

Some strong motivators exist for mothers to RTW, especially if their career is in a satisfactory state, and important for one or both parents. In the meantime, the mother might be under significant stress if she has ambivalence toward co-providing, worry about the relationship equality if she decides to become a "home maker", or diminished confidence about getting back to work after a long leave. One's solution will therefore vary from person to person, in terms of what might be discouraging them from RTW. Here we will discuss some work options that may help the mother stay in the work force or achieve some work-life balance (something that cannot be achieved merely by attaining job options) ...

One can take several steps toward work-life balance after having a baby. The first option is to return to the same job with the same employer. This is the model that many mothers prefer initially, since it makes for a transition back to a familiar routine, especially if one finds their working conditions harmonious. Some people find the benefits provided by the employer too good to pass up on, and most people would prefer to avoid the hassle of going through a job search and interviews. With all this in mind, most of the strategies suggested herein pertain to the same employer.

Changes to the way you interact with your current job environment:

You may be completely fine returning to your same job, without any changes or accommodations. Still, before disregarding this section, consider the changes you can apply to the way you work. These changes are for people who would like to create some head space and not get carried away with work responsibilities after their RTW. You also need to be clear about your boundaries, and able to assertively (not aggressively) express your needs. We will talk more about assertiveness in a later chapter.

The strategies we will discuss here are all about creating a manageable work pace for yourself, as well as using your break times for just that -- to take a break. I have included a a small-step guide to getting into action in the "Initial Plan Guideline" section.

Some items for achieving a manageable work pace are: negotiating realistic deadlines, declining some of your workload/projects, and creating do-not-disturb work periods for yourself.

In addition, expressing to your employer and colleagues (directly or indirectly) that you prefer to only work within formal work hours will be a life saver after RTW. For starters, this calls for directly getting the word out that you have to decline certain work-related requests and trips because you need to make time for your family outside of regular working hours. Insisting that clients and colleagues be on time for their appointments with you and ending your meetings and work days at the predetermined time will also drive home the message. So-called "urgent" matters pertaining to work never truly end, and are therefore better resolved during actual work hours, when you are your most focused, and when everyone else is available to connect with.

Changes to your times and place of work:

To be clear, we are not going into changing your job or the company you work for. Following are some options for carving out more time and space for your family and yourself without changing where you work.

The first option is negotiating "flex time" with your employer. This may take many shapes, but the most common one is coming earlier so as to leave earlier, or vice versa. Many workplaces offer this option to their employees, formally or informally. Also, many mothers have established a relationship with their employers whereby they can take time off during their work days, with the agreement that they will make up those hours later on.

Two other common approaches are working part-time or telecommuting, or a combination of both. In these instances, the employer needs to be assured that your work quality, colleagues, and clients will not suffer from this change – and may even stand to benefit. Some of the mothers who've taken the part-time route report that they do double the work in half the time, just to preserve the new schedule format. As a result, employers usually find themselves getting a better deal with this plan, yet it bears noting that they might not go along with the part-time/telecommuting options at the outset if they do not trust the employee. It goes without saying that not allowing your work to leak into your personal and family time is highly important amid these special arrangements. Meanwhile, bear in mind that a part-time work schedule does not always equal part-time responsibility. Just the same, starting small and building up is generally a healthy alternative to diving right into the deep end of the pool.

Job-sharing is another option, but usually a dreaded accommodation, both on the part of the employer/supervisor and the colleagues. Still, ways exist to shift this attitude, perhaps by highlighting how a colleague or superior might benefit from the new arrangement. As an example, if one of your co-workers is interested in some aspect of your job or clients, this could be their chance to try their hand in it or get more in-depth information. Your supervisor may also see this as a way for you to train someone else for your position, particularly if you are planning to move (upward, downward, or laterally) within or outside the company. Likewise, job-sharing could also be an opportunity for you to see if you might prefer to work in someone else's department/position. Accordingly, the job-sharing desire of other employees is something to be on the lookout for within the company, if this option is of interest to you.

Changes to the work:

As an additional option, you can apply for another job within the company which will give you more head space and time for your personal life. As indicated before, this position can be in any direction (upward, downward, lateral). One thing to consider when entering this territory is whether you want this change permanently or only for a select period of time. It will not always be possible to know as much from the start, but it is important to bear in mind that it may take time and effort to get back to your original position if/when you have a change of heart.

In general, the above option is most applicable when none of the previously mentioned adjustments will suffice or be possible, for one reason or another.

If you are considering new work with the same employer, note that your abilities will fall under consideration, complete with transferable skills to the new position, and that some on-the-job training may be required.

We will not get into the topics of looking for a new job or building your own business herein, since they both deserve a more comprehensive approach.

c. You Will Need Support

You may have had the assumption that you alone are responsible for developing a successful return to work plan. As I mentioned before, however, this process will affect your whole family, complete with your spouse and kids (along with even your extended family and "work family"), all of whom will definitely be involved in the planning phase.

In this chapter, then, I will urge you to think about your relationships and resources. Truth be told, your relationships and resources are what stand to "make or break" you during your RTW process.

Your relationship with yourself:

Let's start at the core. You yourself have a distinct attitude toward life and its challenges. Chances are you have quite a bit of insight into your own strong and weak points, but these can be quite hard to recognize or articulate without a benchmark with which to compare and contrast yourself. One time-tested way of gaining clarity is by asking trusted friends for constructive feedback. Another way is by taking character tests. Granted, such tests offer mere glimpses to our true natures, and there are many of them out there. I think the most comprehensive answer might be found by taking the Myers Briggs Personality test. Keep in mind that the results are not written in stone, and you may find yourself in different categories in different stages in your life.

For the purpose of the RTW process, it is important to

know if you get worried, discouraged, overwhelmed easily, or tend to become inflexible or have unrealistic expectations under stress. This knowledge is valuable when it comes to putting contingency plans in place.

For example, if one has a tendency to over-commit (either to one's family or at work), one needs to develop recognition of how this habit is affecting her. Everyone has their reasons for doing things, including things that may be deemed "bad" habits and attitudes; they all serve or benefit the person in some way, or at least did at some point in time. Therefore, the aim is not to merely put down and criticize that part of ourselves that over-commits. On the contrary, we would be wise to understand the circumstances surrounding this behavior, and approach ourselves with empathy. We should look into what kind of benefits we are deriving from our habits. We are also advised to look into how these habits are not serving our lives in the present situation, where we have to juggle kids, family, work, and who knows what else.

Only after considering the circumstances surrounding such habits in a well-rounded manner, making room for things both good and bad, can a woman start to build a contingency plan. A plan that will help her to keep the benefits while helping her to steer away from the negatives. The first step is looking into the situations that lead to over-commitment, and forming a plan to keep away from those settings, or, if possible, avoid their formation in the first place. This is not an easy feat, as our negative characteristics are very hard to spot in the first place, let alone classify as problematic. Likewise, sometimes changing habits calls for changing social patterns, and taking ourselves out of the crowd we are used to operating in may leave us feeling like the odd one out. While this might call for literally leaving people out of your life at times, it's mostly a matter of not subscribing to the same belief system in terms of how one should live their life, conduct their relationships, or conduct oneself at work.

Your relationship with your baby:

In the midst of your preexisting attitude toward life, you may have found yourself becoming more sensitive about certain issues during the perinatal period.

For example, if you had a hard time getting pregnant and/ or navigating your pregnancy and birth, the effect that these experiences had on you needs to be recognized and accounted for. Meanwhile, regarding the kind of bond you were able to build with your infant, it's useful to take into account whether the care demands were manageable for you. This is not only a matter of assessing how demanding the baby is, but also finding out how you cope with attending to another person, complete with all the intensity doing so requires.

How you feel about yourself as a mother, and about your career after motherhood, has a significant effect on RTW planning. Some mothers recognize how important their careers are to their identities, and some recognize that they would rather become stay-at-home moms. Depending upon where you land on the spectrum, you will arrive at different choices regarding your commitment to work and home, and even what you would look for in a caretaker.

Relationships with husband, parents, in-laws, professional colleagues, employer, supervisor, clients, & peers

Yes, it does take a village to raise a child, even if your fellow villagers never set a hand upon your baby. One can easily identify the ways in which a mother would struggle without financial or emotional security, but beyond these factors, many mothers still struggle with just getting from one day to the next...

We all hold vastly different family support expectations, as well as need levels when it comes to being understood. All in all, though, it's taxing to see how many mothers judge themselves for having difficulty managing all their responsibilities, especially when they seemingly "have it all" (financial, emotional, and social support) and yet are "still complaining." Yet it pays to be mindful of the fact that someone else's struggle, no matter how big it may be (or seem to be), does not negate the struggle of a mother who has more support. In the same way that you would acknowledge something basic like being hungry, you can also acknowledge less traditionally urgent needs, such as requiring more space, time, or support to manage motherhood, without a fear of seeming petty or difficult. After all, every household operates differently:

Some mothers would not even think to ask their partners for help with the laundry, while others would simply expect such help as a part of their partnership deal. Some require more privacy in the bathroom than others, often waiting to use it after the kids are asleep, or making the point that bathroom time is off limits, and the children are prohibited from knocking on the door.

In general, how is your support network responding to your changing needs and perception of what constitutes support after motherhood?

A lot of talking points apply here. Do you have a friend (or parent, husband, or counselor) with whom to talk about such points? As discussed, it often makes a big difference when you can hash things out with a good listener whom you trust, which brings us to our next topic...

What resources are available to you? Go down the list and take stock of what you have to work with, and, of course, discuss it with those you trust:

- Financial ability to afford adequate daycare, house cleaners, and other third-party support systems
- Friends and family who are willing to help
- Daycare that is satisfactory to the mother's standards (location, caretakers etc.)
- Mother's occupation (assess rigidity of working hours and workload)
- Father's occupation (assess rigidity of working hours and workload)

d. Detailed Plan and Guidelines

Detailed Plan:

Following are the basic questions you need to address in a family context before returning to work.

- What days/hours are you working?
- Who will be providing care while you work? When, where, and how?
- What are the logistics of meal preparation?
- Who is dropping the children off regularly? (What about when regular caretakers are not available?)
- Will the woman have any time for herself? When, where, and how?
- What else is on your plate? (Moving, renovations, financial goals and challenges…)
- How will you approach managing the above issues? Verbal planning? Written planning? Who is central to the plan-making?
- What forms of support do you have? Can you bring in more support?
- What are the contingency plans when the first-tier plans fall through?

Guidelines

Following are four essential points to consider before returning to work.

1.   Practice your day before returning to work:

Think of this as a rehearsal that will save you a lot of headaches when you actually return. Ideally, start practicing at least two weeks ahead of time, so that you will have one extra week to smooth out any issues that might come up in the first week. Put all your players (nanny, grandparents, husband, neighbors, etc.) on the game board. Things will not be perfect upon your return, but at least you will know what to expect upon going in again. Meanwhile, note that a mother can always expect some part of her brain to be wrapped up in what may be going on with her kids when she is not around, but the rehearsal period will allow preparation for that, as well. So be sure to practice everything, from waking up to being away from kids, to pumping, to meal preparations and going to bed on time. When you are out of the house to practice, you can also actually visit your workplace, check in with your supervisor and colleagues, and catch up on the office agenda. While you're at it, don't hesitate to daydream and even go to a movie for a change.

2.   Put your new priorities to work

You have now been through the initial months of motherhood, and whether or not you are looking forward to getting back to work or wishing you could stay home, your worldview has definitely changed. Most new mothers become sharply aware of their priorities, whether or not those priorities have shifted on a basic level. Some things that you were once able to let linger, take on as a favor, or devote gradually unfolding time to are now harder to tolerate. Your time and your focus are now more valuable commodities than ever before, and as such you will become more selective about where you direct them. If you are resistant to the natural change, and still wanting to be everywhere for everyone, or are having a hard time turning down requests, your life will become even less manageable after you RTW. Accordingly, set priorities that *work for you*, rather than making you work.

3. Put things into action

One can think, talk, and plan forever, but the basic rule of putting things into action is *acting* on them. To bring ideas into action, act – take the leap. It is not and never will be possible to plan everything before we dive onto the action field. Only then will you be able to test your willingness and ability to take the necessary steps to reach your desired destination. You will also become aware of alternative paths that may lead to similarly desired results. It is not easy to see the opportunities within a field before becoming personally familiar with that field, in addition to experiencing how you interact with the other people on it.

Your plan needn't even be complete before you act. You can figure out the remainder of the plan, and how to respond to challenges, while you are in action. Don't wait for conditions to become perfect, as they never will be.

I would like you to put the following practice into action, today: Approach even the smallest activity, from remembering to floss your teeth three times a day to reminding yourself to not end your sentences at a higher pitch, as if you are asking a question, for the next 30 days. The largest activity you include in this process needs to be something that starts and finishes in 30 days, no longer. You may know this much quoted sequence from thoughts to destiny...

"Your beliefs become your thoughts,
Your thoughts become your words,
Your words become your actions,
Your actions become your habits,
Your habits become your values,
Your values become your destiny."
—Mahatma Gandhi

For the next 30 days, take the smallest step you can manage to create new habits. Note that my encouragement to act is not an invitation to be hasty or impulsive, but to shed whatever habit, fear, or form of reluctance is inhibiting you from taking the initial steps toward shaping your world.

4. You do not have the luxury of not taking care of yourself

Here's a valuable question: "Who will take care of everything you are taking care of AND you when you cannot get out of bed?" It is prudent to discuss this matter with some friends and family members, and to keep their contact information handy in the event of Plan B. Many women find it hard to get such help, or to even get time off for sick days, even in tightly-knit families. The basics of self-care include sleeping at least seven and a half hours a day, eating at least three meals a day (including vegetables and protein), having time to unwind and feel supported, and having time to connect with family and friends. With these basics in tow, you can stay on top of your game, and even have the stamina to run in all different directions with minimal outside support.

e. Self Care

N.E.S.T.S +

The oft-used acronym NESTS, well-known among caretakers, stands for Nutrition, Exercise, Sleep, Time for self, and Social support. These are the basic components of self-care for any individual to lead a healthy life, both physically and mentally (which are inseparable). A stable mind is founded on a healthy body; a healthy body depends upon a stable mind.

I have added one additional point to this acronym (Train your focus and willpower) to highlight the fact that habitual negative thinking leaves us distressed and lifeless, and will eventually erode our physical health, as well.

Nutrition

Recommended Dietary Women Allowance	19 – 50 years		
	Non-pregnant	Pregnant	Breastfeeding
Folate (mcg/day)	400	600	500
Iron (mg/day)	18	27	9
Vitamin A (mcg RAE/day)	700	770	1300
Vitamin C (mg/day)	75	85	120
Vitamin D (mcg/day)	5	5	5

Calcium (mg/day)	**1000**	**1000**	**1000**
Zinc (mg/day)	8	11	12
Vitamin B6 (mg/day)	1.3	1.9	2.0
Magnesium (mg/day)	310 *(19 - 30 y)* 320 *(31 – 50 y)*	350 *(19 - 30 y)* 360 *(31 – 50 y)*	310 *(19 - 30 y)* 320 *(31 – 50 y)*
Vitamin B12 (mcg/day)	2.4	2.6	2.8

Nutrient amounts in bold font indicate an Adequate Intake (AI)
Taken from Health Canada Prenatal Nutrition Guidelines for Professionals

Exercise

At minimum, you should be sure not to remain seated for more than one hour. On a more intensive level, exercising 3 to 5 times per week, 45 to 60 minutes at a time, hitting 50 to 80 percent of your maximum heart-rate (if doing aerobics) across a span of 12 weeks stands to enhance not only your physical health, but your mental health profile. This level of exercise regime is indeed recommended for combating Major Depressive Disorder (MDD). Note that aerobic workouts are particularly effective. Also, even if you cannot reach or maintain the level of working out that I'm recommending here, a sincere and sustained commitment to exercise can only help you.

Sleep (hygienic)

We need to sleep for at least seven and a half hours a day, as not getting enough sleep is the utmost contributor to poor mood and mental health during your initial post-partum months. Sleepless nights and unstable moods are to be expected from both parents for about a year, but more so in the initial six months. Meanwhile, the parents' relationship will also go through a rocky period in the first two years after having a baby. The level of marital satisfaction declines, but couples usually emerge with a better understanding of each other, and so their relationship dynamic is strengthened via trial by fire.

While attending to your baby will undoubtedly reduce your ability to get a full night's sleep, some measures exist to help you make the best of your situation. The term "sleep hygiene" refers to practices that are necessary for having normal, quality nighttime sleep, as well as daytime alertness.

The most important sleep hygiene measure is to maintain a regular wake-and-sleep pattern, seven days a week. It is also important to spend an appropriate amount of time in bed – not too little, nor too much. During the first six months of a baby's life, this will not be a perfect schedule. It is very important that you do not compare your and your baby's schedule against that of others, much less something prescribed by a book. Be very patient and forgiving with yourself, and remember that getting used to how things are or carrying out seemingly simple tasks may take more time than you thought they would.

In general, napping throughout the day is discouraged when it comes to sleep hygiene, but you are strongly encouraged to do so post-partum, every time you get the chance, whether it be day or night. Refer to the sleep diary at the appendix for some practices that may be helpful.

Time for Yourself

This means something different for everyone. Initially, many mothers cannot decide if they need time for themselves or just more sleep. Sleep tends to win, especially if you are getting less than 4 hours a day.

As for "proper" time for yourself, it can mean professional development, coffee with friends, or even pampering time…

Social Support (Tend and Befriend)

It has been discovered that it is not the existence of stress but the belief that stress is bad for you that is detrimental to your health.

Likewise, oxytocin is secreted during times of distress, which promotes the will to connect with others for support. If we do connect with others during times of distress, and get the support we're looking for, we ultimately get the physical benefits of the initial oxytocin release, which helps to recover the damaged cells in our body (i.e., heart muscles) that stemmed from the initial stress. In this way, stress has ultimately positive potential.

Recall the last time you felt all alone in dealing with a responsibility, or a challenge in your life. Did you reach out to someone, either to gain support for the task itself or to open up about your anxiety? Life's challenges exist for everyone, and we feel more motivated to grapple with them if we know that someone is and will be there for us. When we know that someone we trust has our back, the world can change from a cold and scary place to one of excitement and adventure. So pick and choose your allies with care.

Never forget: You do not have to do it on your own. There is no point in draining yourself by trying to figure everything out on your own. Who else can help you find your way? Pick and choose from the people in your life, and add new ones as necessary. These people can be elders, mentors, other mothers who have been there before, and maybe even your niece, nephew, or neighbor, who can watch your kids while you take a quick and much-needed shower. If you do not have, or never have had, an actual mentor, then researching mentoring options and environments has the potential to open up a lot of doorways.

Join groups, also, preferably in the physical world. You need to concentrate on and focus your energies toward devising your own optimum strategy. Spend time with people that empower and trust you. Discuss and revise your action plan(s) with them.

Train your focus and will power (radio)

Oftentimes, we live oblivious to the fact that our attention can be tuned and fine-tuned like a radio. Something comes to our mind, and we follow the train of the idea, the thought, until we get distracted by something else. It is one thing if the thought pertains to our immediate surroundings or circumstances; i.e., figuring out a way to get back into the house when you are locked out. Such is a practical issue in pressing need of a resolution. It is another thing, though, if you randomly start to remember all the negative things people have said about you, or times when others have questioned your ability to do anything right. (Both of which are linked together, as thoughts tend to be...)

It's worth bearing in mind that it is not what happens to us, but how we look at it, that determines whether or not something is stressful. Many people get locked out of their homes, cars, drawers, accounts, and computers, but our responses to these challenges differ. Our differing upbringings, living situations, and access to resources lead to differing reactions to external circumstances. We cannot make generalizations about which conditions bring which results, because even the most comfortable minds can be prone to depression, whereas people from war-torn families can bear the determination to live a full and happy life, and so on. It is our ability to be the "boss" of our own minds that makes the difference.

Accordingly, if you become aware that a certain thought is eating you up, interrupt it. Turn your attention to another channel. We keep trying to think our way out of (often old) hurts and fears. We try to protect ourselves from falling into the same situations that we regret from our past in our future. However, at all junctures, some answers cannot be accessed through basic thought, and some things – many things – are not in our control. Yet we easily spiral into trying to find a way out of them.

Try responding to thoughts that deplete your energy the same way as a mother would when she sees her kids struggling – by intervening in a positive way. Emulate a parent, friend, mentor, or counselor who you've seen carrying out such intervention. Above all else, the key is to STOP and redirect your focus to something that lightens your heart and gives you strength. This can even be external: your children or family, nature or God. Nurture the attitude that you've done your best, and you are leaving the problem in their hands for the time being.

Resources Regarding Exercise:

http://www.ncbi.nlm.nih.gov/pubmed/15626549
http://psychcentral.com/news/2013/05/11/new-guidelines-for-using-exercise-as-an-antidepressant/54728.html

Regarding Sleep:

https://sleepfoundation.org/sleep-diary/SleepDiaryv6.pdf
https://sleepfoundation.org/ask-the-expert/sleep-hygiene/page/0/1

*The not napping during the day comment in this sleep hygiene article is not appropriate for new mothers who should take a nap whenever they can in the first months!!!

Social Support:

http://www.ncbi.nlm.nih.gov/pmc/articles/PMC3374921/
http://www.ncbi.nlm.nih.gov/pmc/articles/PMC3410434/
http://www.ncbi.nlm.nih.gov/pmc/articles/PMC3780662/
http://www.apa.org/monitor/feb08/oxytocin.aspx
http://www.eurekaselect.com/99865/article
http://www.ted.com/talks/kelly_mcgonigal_how_to_make_stress_your_friend?language=en

f. Prepare The Workplace for Your Return

If, before you left your workplace, you did not make it ready for your return, do not worry. Begin the process by contacting your employer at least two months before you go back to work, and prepare them for your return. Note that whether or not you are already employed, your ultimate career destiny should not be a pressing concern at this time; it is far wiser and healthier to take things one step at a time. Indeed, during this initial phase of activity, one important benefit can be the return or establishment of your self-confidence...

In general, the workplace has a strong commitment to work and life balance.

For the most part, employers would like to keep their employees and clients happy. Doing so just makes for good business. If you have an employer that openly declares their commitment to work-life balance, then now is a good time for them to make good on that commitment.

This is among the issues you want to open up for conversation with your supervisor or employer before you leave to give birth and take care of your baby. It is relatively easy to learn about a company's official policy, but takes a little more attentiveness to understand their actual culture. To be sure, an authentic workplace culture, one which not only regards the needs of new mothers, but even new fathers and those who care for aging parents, always has an advantage in terms of retaining and satisfying employees. You may already have an idea of your colleague's opinions regarding maternity leave and returning to work, but making your own expectations and requirements explicit will save you a lot of anxiety and headaches when it comes time for your return. The hardship here is that most mothers, unless they are not first-time mothers, have a hard time envisioning the realities of what they will need upon returning to work. In such cases, making a point of talking to some colleagues and friends that have been through the same hassle is paramount.

Suitable modified work arrangements.

One does not show up and dive right into work on one's first day back. Neither the employee nor the employer find starting "cold turkey" to be easy, much less desirable. Many others ways of tipping your toes back into the work environment exist. (Note, however, that even before you return, it's always wise to be up-to-date on the technology, news, and relevant networking happenings pertaining to your field, by way of LinkedIn and other professional communication tools.)

For example, you can either negotiate a Gradual Return To Work or use your vacation or other available days off to schedule one for yourself.

For those who aren't familiar with Gradual RTWs; they are just as they sound. You and your employers agree on a plan, arranging a schedule of the tasks you will be responsible for, one wherein you gradually increase your number of days/hours at the office, or maintain a steady time schedule yet steadily widen the scope of your work tasks.

The most common modified work arrangement for mothers consists of flexible hours (a very common desire nowadays, alongside of being able to explore one's job options). They may commit to a certain amount of hours-per-week or project finish dates, and they reach their goals across non-standard work hours.

You can even start two days a week, and then increase your presence by one day every week. You may also go in for half-days at times. You can arrange your precise plan according to your specific needs, and you will find that many employers will be open to discussing GRTW, so long as they are convinced that they are getting your full commitment to work when you are on company time.

Someone has the responsibility to coordinate Return to Work.

Even if the company does not have an assigned employee tasked with managing Return To Work, you might wish to "assign" a person yourself. The ability to do so will exist hand-in-hand with your skills in terms of networking and using social media, for the stronger you are here, the more people will be in your corner. Your coordinator will ideally be someone who has an interest and invested stake in your successful return: a supervisor, perhaps, or HR personnel member who has previous experience with Returning To Work issues.

The identity of this person needs to be determined, and all pertinent details discussed, before your maternity leave begins. Talk with them to establish the basics, such as their agreement to support your RTW process, the options available to you, and their ideas on creating contingency plans. It is too early to know exactly what head-space and life situations will characterize your return, so making rigid plans is not an option at this juncture.

The employer or you must make early and considerate contact to communicate about the Return To Work process.

Do not wait for people to remember your return dates, nor know the full extent of your needs. Take the initiative of visiting your workplace with your baby, the better to show your employer and colleagues what you have been working on (i.e., having and raising a child) for your stretch of absence. Allow them to also attain more context in terms of your mood and new daily schedule, which revolves around your little one. This not only allows your colleagues to re-establish personal contact with you, it encourages them to be more tolerant when you have to attend to your baby's last-minute needs.

If you do not let them see what your life looks like right now, your employers and supervisors will not viscerally understand what you are going through, and will thus be more likely to question your work commitment and ethic. So make that contact, be it at work itself or during a lunch visit. This will also give you a chance to learn about the latest work events and projects, and open up a discussion regarding where you will fit and what you will start working on when you return.

Carry out a thorough discussion regarding the modifications' effect on coworkers and work flow.

Modifications pertaining to your work schedule or task flow may be a major source of concern to you and your supervisors alike. The most important point here is that all parties be open to finding effective solutions. Otherwise, work environments can grow quickly toxic. It is never desirable to continue working with a disgruntled colleague, supervisor, or employer.

So the real challenge here is connecting with your point of contact in a way that inspires them to ensure a win-win situation. Open and ongoing communication among the involved parties is the only way to preserve a healthy and mutually beneficial arrangement.

A short note: A win-win situation is one wherein the parties involved give each other time and space to understand and express their needs. Usually, conflicts arise because parties come to think that their needs clash with each other, but the truth is that each person has *differing* needs, not necessarily clashing ones. Once you discover this, getting everybody's needs met is a breeze.

4. After Returning to Work

Give yourself some time to get used to the new routine.

Three months is the average time that it takes most women to adjust. Not only do you adjust, but all the various puzzle pieces pertaining to you settle into place in around three months. Many women expect all to be settled in the first week, and feel panic and despair when this does not pan out. Note that anxiety is best not viewed as a problem at this time; it is in fact welcome, because it can motivate us to get our tasks in order. But judging yourself for feeling anxious – and thinking that none of the other, "proper" mothers are going through these kinds of issues – will lead you to start feeling despair, which itself is detrimental for coming up with solutions.

Contingency Planning

Contingency planning can also be called the Management Stage. After you are back at work, this planning process comes about naturally. We create Plan B and Plan C and beyond, comparing and contrasting the benefits and challenges of each. Below I will spell out this process and make its assorted aspects explicit. Note that visual decision-making tools are very helpful when it comes to management...

What worked; what did not work?

Contingency planning is a circular process, insofar as it involves trial, error, and revision, but we can say that it starts with maintenance.

While maintaining our array of tasks and schedules, we analyze what is working, what is not working, and what can be done better.

Modifications to plans.

If we decide that some things are not working or need to be taken care of in a different, better way, then it's at this point when we start generating solution ideas. At this stage, you may already have some solutions lined up, or you may have to go back to the drawing board. If doing so is relevant to your situation, create a cut-and-pasted "problems, solutions, negatives, and positives" board, which will allow you to get the lay of the land. You can also draw up charts or pictures, or start to journal without editing yourself. This will all support the brainstorming-without-editing-yourself stage. We avoid making linear, concrete lists at this stage, because we want to tap into our right brain, which offers seemingly infinite ways of coming up with new ideas.

The process is open-ended.

We do not stop finding new ways of doing things or solutions to the problems that we face. Likewise, we can put our ideas and solutions to the test only by implementing them. Always remember that we can better understand the terrain and generate more options while we are in motion, rather than merely thinking about solutions to our roadblocks from a sedentary vantage point.

Ongoing monitoring:

Are we doing things right?

Such is the question that most often gets us thinking about our contingency plans. We monitor whether we are happy with the fruits of our efforts, in accordance with our original plan. If we are not getting what we need, discomfort will begin to set in. At that point, we wonder about better ways of reaching our goals: "Can I be faster? More meticulous in planning? Can I get more help? Who can help me with this? Can I ask my partner to do things differently?" And so on...

Are we doing the right things?

We test out our various ideas by putting them to use, and we keep putting them to use as long as they serve their purpose. Unless your mindset resembles an airtight bureaucracy (which is not uncommon), you may at times find yourself asking if you want to be doing what you're doing. Such is when your goals start to change. Even without us realizing it, oftentimes our life priorities change. Before we had children, our work and personal life were very important to us, but now perhaps providing for your family and spending more time with your children is your focus. Attaining a satisfying work-family balance generally takes a lot of time and requires a lot of patience and practice. Our targets keep moving in accordance with our ever-shifting priorities and life realities. So in this stage, the management stage, we ask, "Am I doing the right things to reap the benefits that I want today?"

My wish for you is all the benefits imaginable

Bibliography

Baxter, J., "Is Money the Main Reason Mothers Return to Work After Childbearing?" *Journal of Population Research* Vol. 25, No.2, (September 2008), pp. 141-160.

Hock, E., Christman, K., Hock, M., "Factors Associated with Decisions About Return to Work in Mothers of Infants" *Developmental Psychology,* Vol. 16, No. 5, (1980), pp. 535-536.

Lee, R. E., "When Midcareer Mothers First Return to Work: Counseling Concerns" *Journal of Counseling and Development* Vol. 63, (September 1984), pp.35-39.

Feldman, R., Sussman, A. L., Zigler, E., "Parental Leave and Work Adaptation at the Transition to Parenthood: Individual, Marital, and Social Correlates" *Applied Developmental Psychology* Vol.25, (2004), pp. 459-479.

About the Author

Evren Suri Westhead is a Registered Clinical Counsellor focusing on Return To The World of Work Counseling with mothers. She holds a Masters Degree in Business Administration. Her approach to therapy is, as she calls it, Experience Therapy, where she values the visceral understanding of her clients more than talk. She is influenced by a variety of disciplines that bring about the desired changes for her clients and keeps herself and her audience up to date with her online expert interviews at workingmother.ca.

www.ingramcontent.com/pod-product-compliance
Lightning Source LLC
Chambersburg PA
CBHW050523290526
45786CB00007B/2669